CAREGIVERS & CLIENTS

Therapeutic Home Arts & Recreation Guide

I0467445

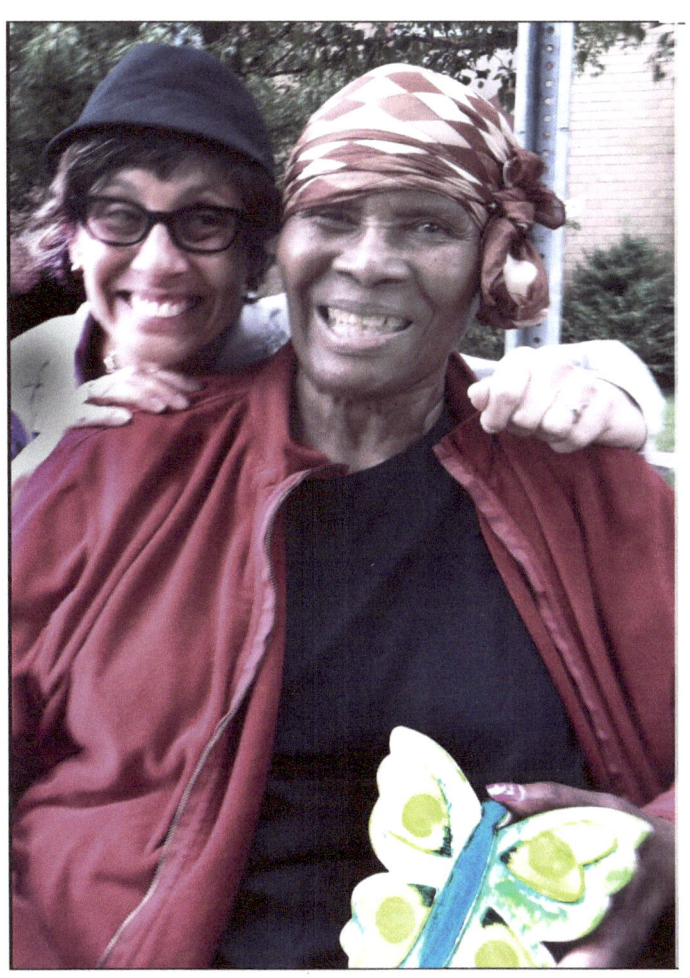

For Milt who became my good friend.

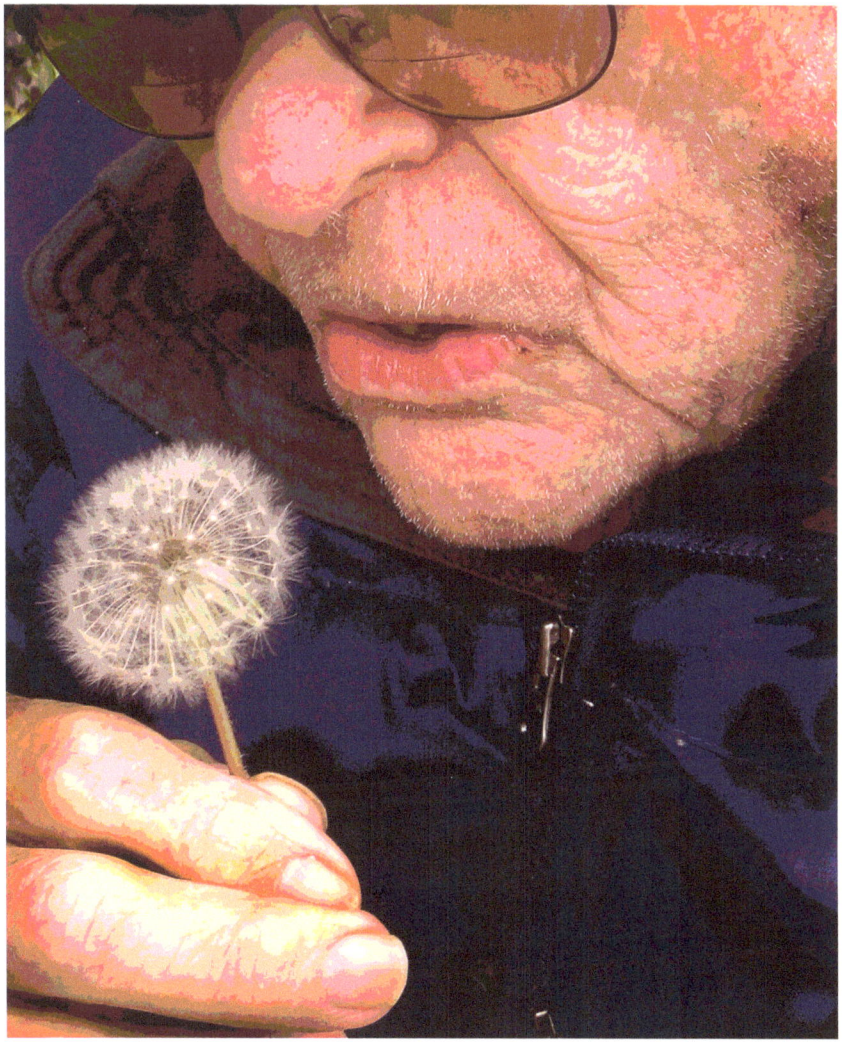

Written and Photographed by Rebecca Singer

2   0   1   4

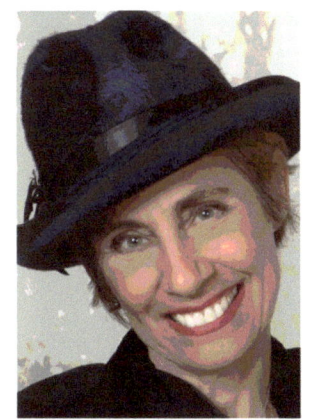

My name is Rebecca Singer.

I have been practicing art since I was a small child. My entire career wraps around art. I have worked as a graphic designer, interior designer and artist.

Over ten years ago, I began working with a group of ladies at the Montifiore Senior Center. They needed an instructor for their sewing group. I worked with this group three times a week for seven years. We created colorful aprons, quilts, bags, dolls and more.

I found great satisfaction being a cheerleader for the group, creating opportunities for them to show their work, and building their skills and confidence along the way. In another group, composed of people who are blind, I prepared sinple sewing projects.

Group Projects

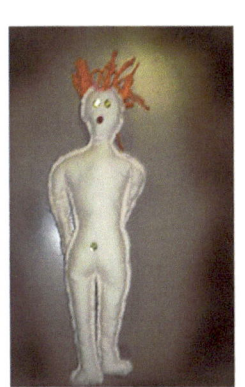

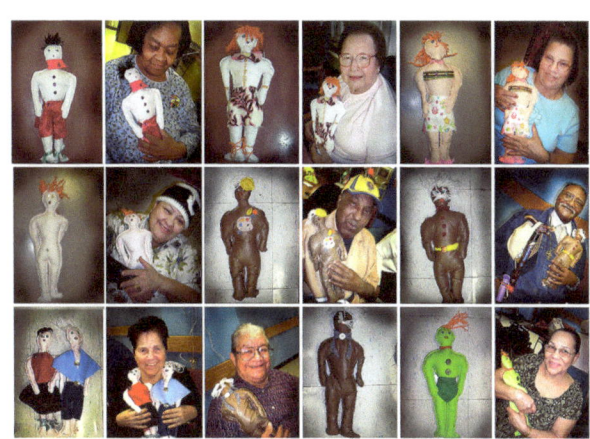

1.

Hat Project

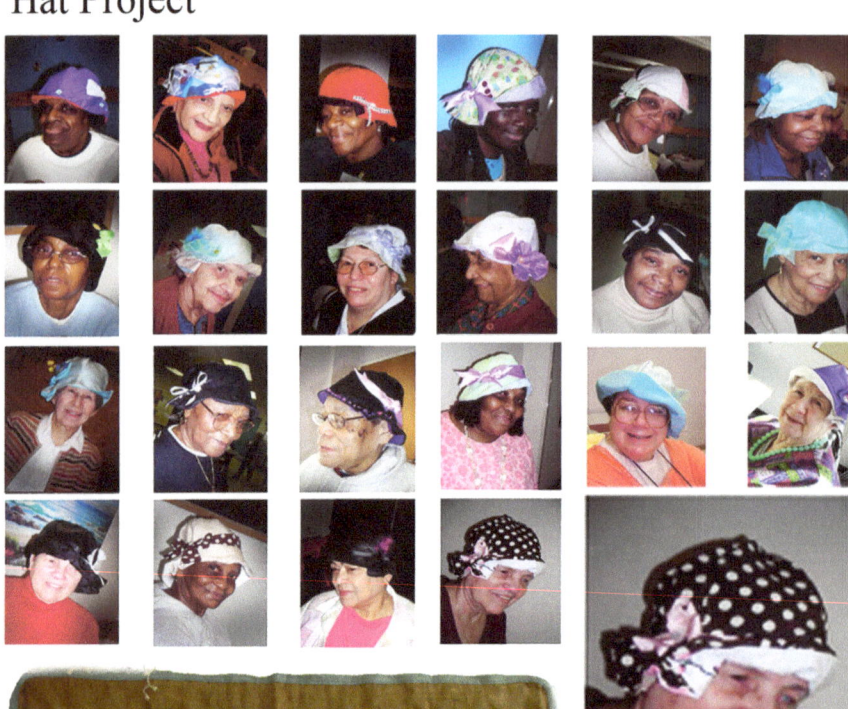

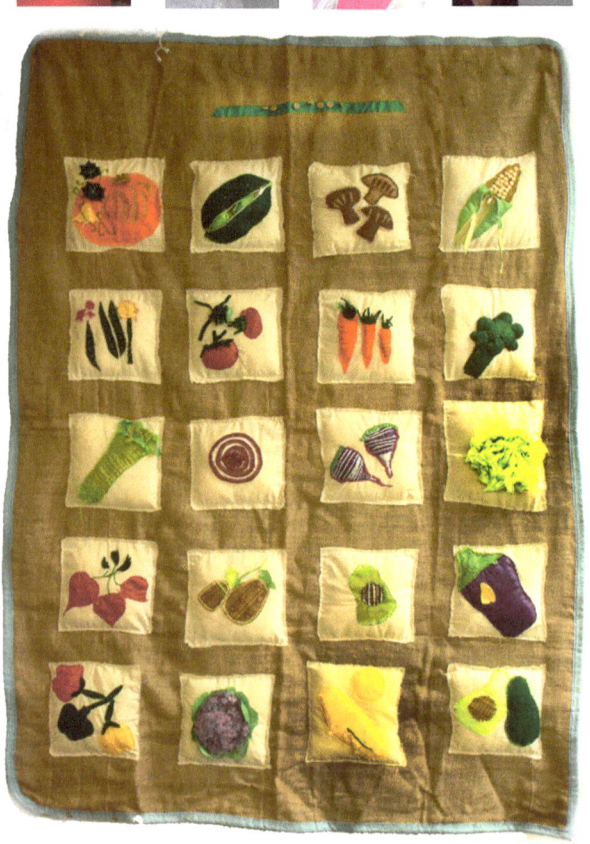

Seniors Go Green Nutrition Quilt

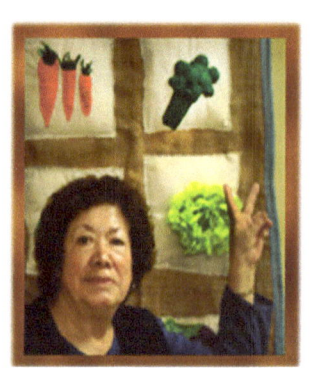

I produce projects with people who have physical problems, psychological issues, and memory challenges. We enjoy working with different materials and producing a finished product. Always hang their work and praise them. This elevates their spirits.

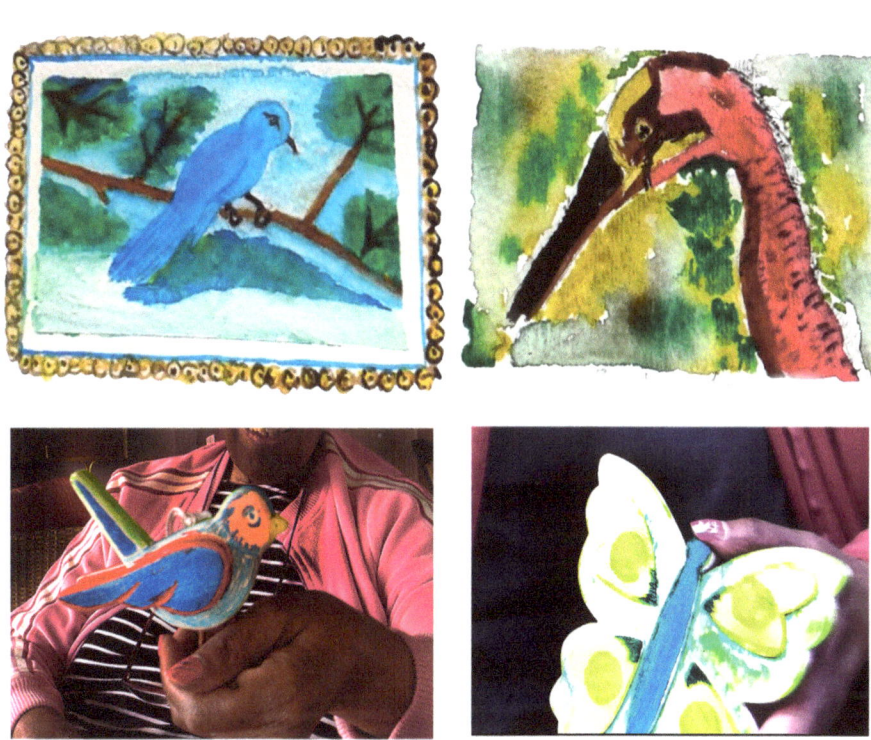

Working One on One

For individual clients I design programs that meet their interests. A retired accountant, responded to *addition flash cards* which brougth back his ability to add and gave him lots of confidence. He spoke very little and no one was sure how much he could speak. So, I tried picture flash cards with him and this over time renewed his ability to speak!

3.

For Home Health Aides and Care Givers

How To Enjoy Your Client
Improve His Health and Yours Too.
Laugh

I never used to laugh. My family always told me that
I was missing the laughter gene. So somehow several
years ago, I taught myself how to laugh. I used any
opportunity to laugh and I noticed it lifted my spirits
and the spirits of those around me. Laugh as much as
you can and you will see that you feel happier and so
do your friends and family.

Words

Find and use words from your client's culture.
For example, if your client speaks Spanish, add "ita"
to their name. It is a sign of affection; Rosa becomes
Rosita, Yolanda becomes Yolandita. If your client
speaks Yiddish, call him a "mench." A "mench" is a
another name for a very good person. Familiar words
make people feel close.   It is as if we are sharing our
own special language and and we have our own special
names.

4.

Food

Learn about the food your client likes. Ask him to tell you how he likes his food cooked. Go to the market that carries the kind of food he likes. If you are the care giver and you are Jamacian, and he is Russian, your taste in food may be very different. Try to see this as an opportunity to to explore different tastes. When you make a meal for yourself, offer some to your client. It's fun to exchange tastes and try new things.

Cook

Make easy foods **with** your client. Soup is fun to make and some vegetables are soft enough to cut with a plastic knife. Fruit salad is also easy to slice. Cookie dough can be rolled and pressed on to a tray and this is great exercise for the hands. The point is to involve your client in every day life.
Everyone likes to feel useful and productive. Lastly, it's fun to share the food you have made. Invite your neighbor to join you. This makes it a party!

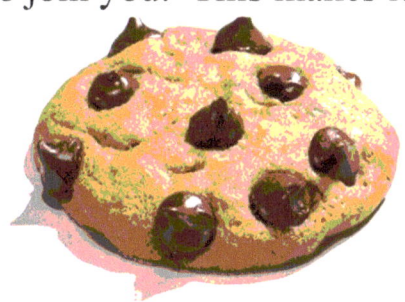

Once my client told me he made great scrambled eggs.
He said he'd like to make them for me.
So I responded, "great, let's make them."
I think he was aftraid he might not be able to. So I
slipped a chair behind him incase he lost his balance
and he did a great job making the eggs.
He felt very proud of himself.

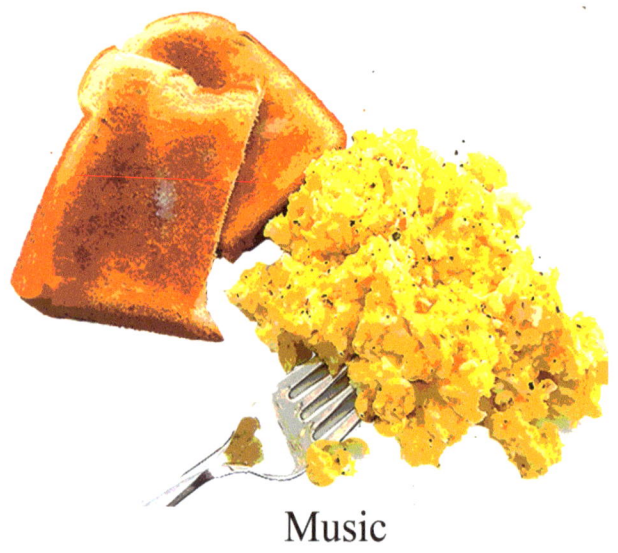

Music

Many seniors like patriotic music. They like Sinatra,
Judy Garland and they like to sing. Singing releases
endorphins which makes us feel happy. So sing
and get them to sing too!
With one client, I learned the Judy Garland
part of a song and he learned the Mickey Rooney
part of the song. We rehearsed it and it became "our"
song.

6.

Create an Event

Once I picked up three different chocolate bars. We invited our neighbor to taste test with us. We each tasted the bars, one at a time, no peaking, letting it dissolve in our mouths and then describing the tastes. At the end, we had to guess which bar was which. It was loads of fun and delicious too. This game of tasting can be done with apples, tea, coffee, licorice and more.

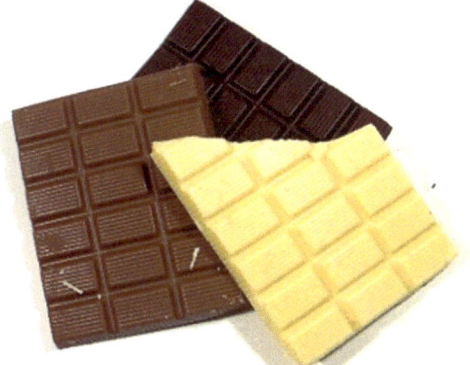

Hair and Clothing

Take your client for a hair cut or help to style their hair. Paint their nails if they are a woman and put on their best clothes. Then go out for coffee and show off! It's been said, "to look good is to feel good!"

Watch Judge Judy

Try to guess which person Judy will pick as the winner. Have a good, hard laugh at the contestants.

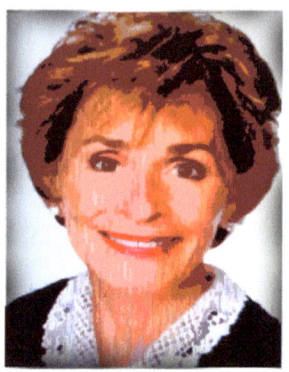

Memory Games

If your client is having trouble remembering words,
Pick up a box of picture flash cards and make a game
of it. Any memory games are great for Seniors.
If you have no flash cards, just make up the game.
For example, say: "Colors, how many colors can we
name?" Or "Let's name cities or states."
Tell your client that you want to keep him sharp and
this is the reason for the games.

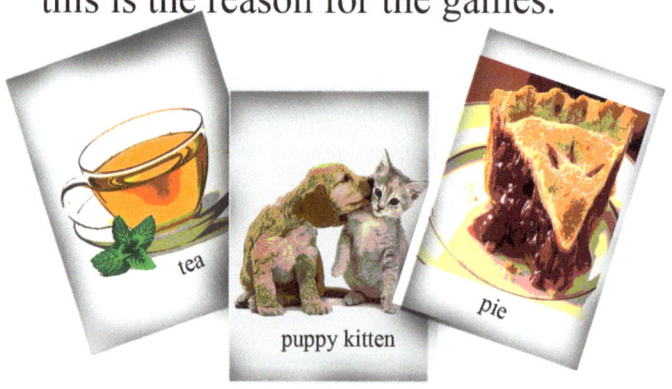

Paint Pictures

Put them on the wall and date it. Do this every week
and see how the paintings change over time.

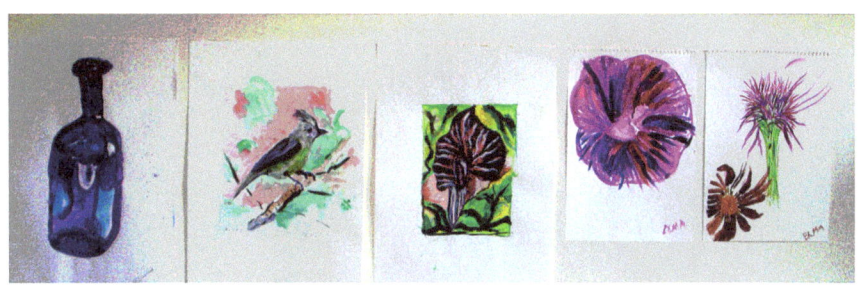

Photography

If you like photography, take pictures of the things you
do and the places you go. Have the local drug store or
photo store print them. It's fun to remember the
places you've gone and things you've done together.
Show your client the pictures and ask them to
remember the event. If you have a photo of yourself,
put it in a prominent place with your name on it.
sometimes your client might need help remembering
your name.

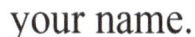

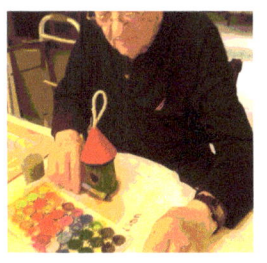
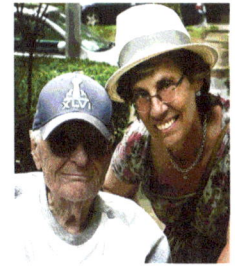

Hug or Hold Hands

Everyone loves affection.

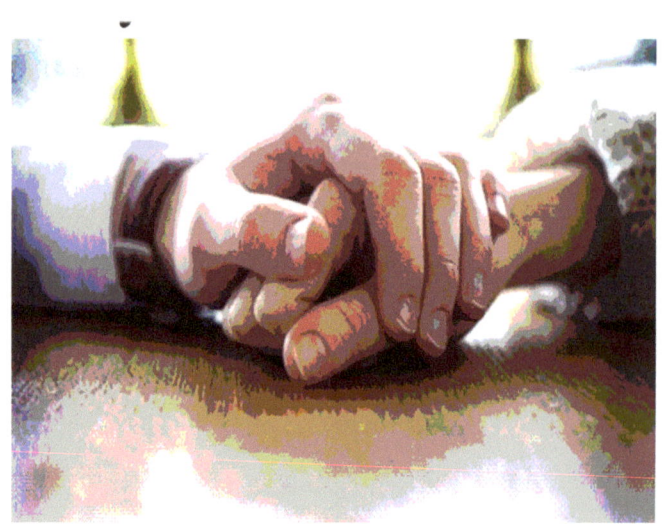

Visit a Flower shop

Enjoy the colors and smells.
Breathe!

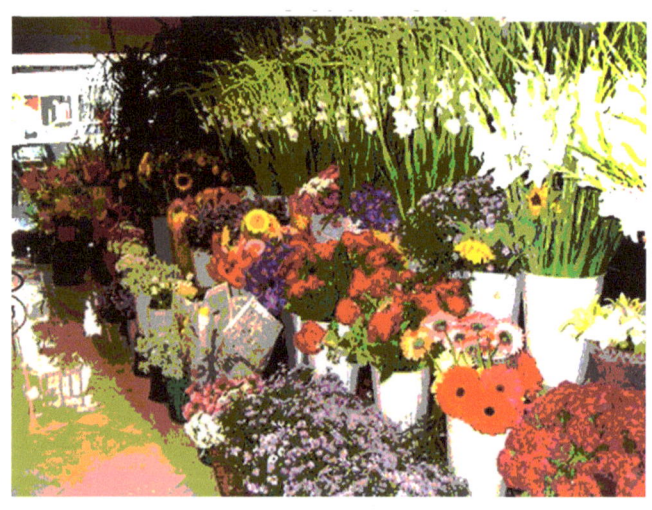

Sunlight

Open the Shades and Enjoy the Light!
The vitamins from the sun are good for us.

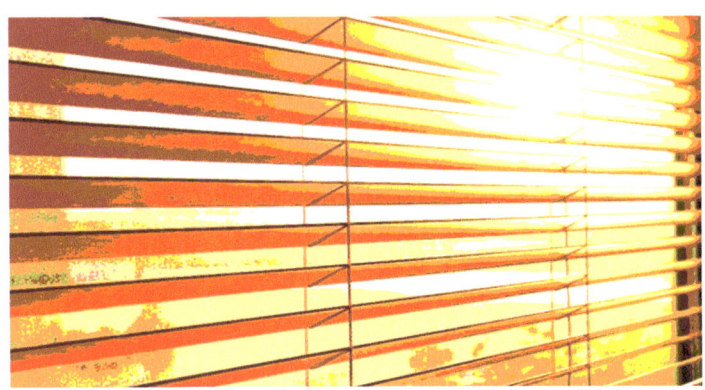

Spa Day

Create a spa day and give your client a neck massage,
then do hair and nails.

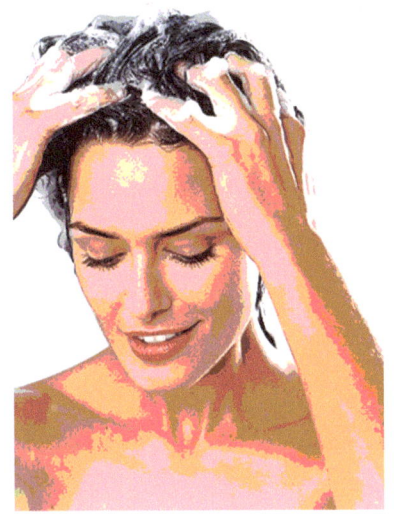

11.

Polish Shoes

Polishing shoes can be very satisfying and
also great exercise for the hands

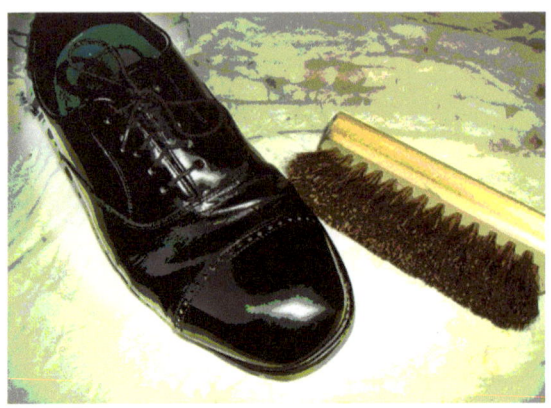

Polish Silver
Everyone loves thje way polished silver looks.
It's great exercise for the hands and very satisfying
as well

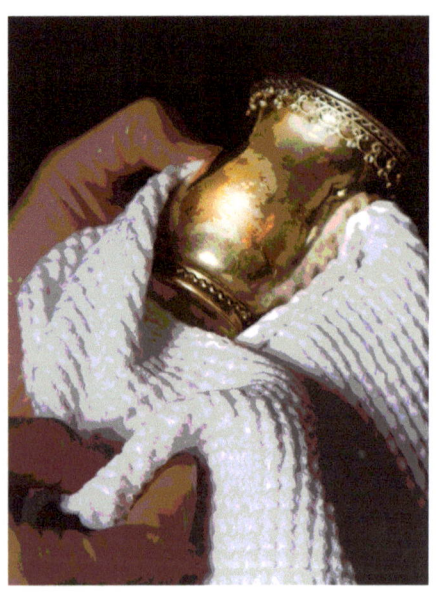

Foot Massage

It seems that a foot massage is also good for other parts of the body. This is known as reflexology. And who doesn't love a good foot massage?

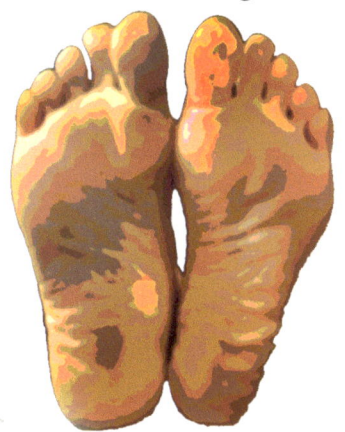

Pet Store Trips

Take your client to the pet store. Puppies are so sweet and hear warming. Birds and fish are wonderful to watch.

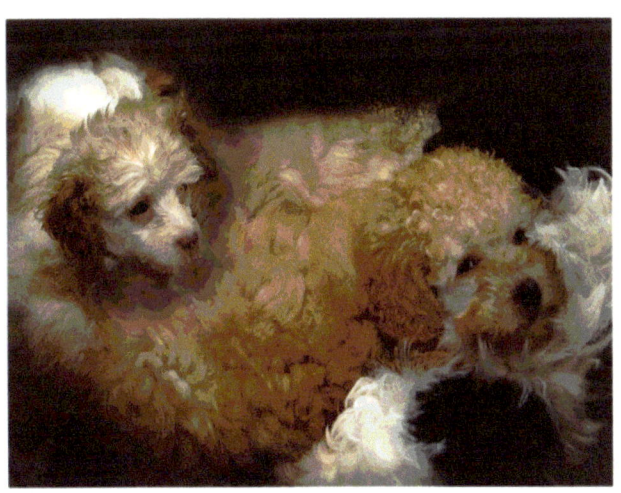

Calender

Make a large weekly calender and put one main event on it for every day. The main event could be as simple as going to the produce market, or going for coffee at the local coffee shop. These small trips are stimulating and create a difference in each day. Let your client help plan the week making sure there are other events besides going to the Doctor.
Try to make the schedule interesting, each day being different. The schedule might look like this:

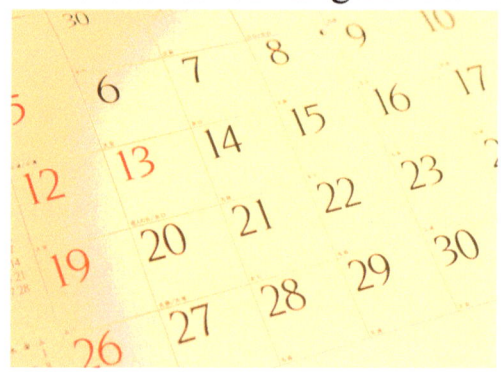

Morning

Have breakfast, get dressed, comb hair, brush teeth, discuss the event that is on the agenda.
Announce the day, date, time, weather. Write it on a large pad that can be seen.

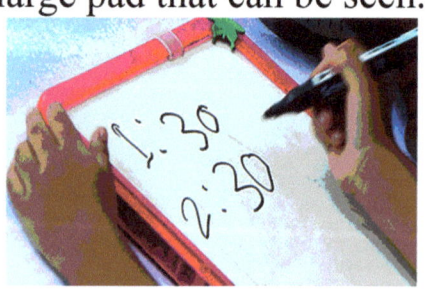

Exercise

Throw a ball or balloon, stretch.
Exercise to music or find a television show
where they are exercising and just follow along.

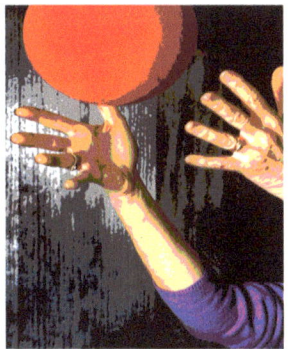

Take a Break

Games

Engage in memory games, such as cards,
or "opposites," for example, you say: "hot"
your client says, :"cold."
Play: "name the cities in the United States."
Over time these games really help keep the
memory sharp.

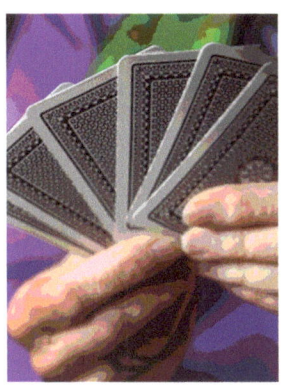

Lunch

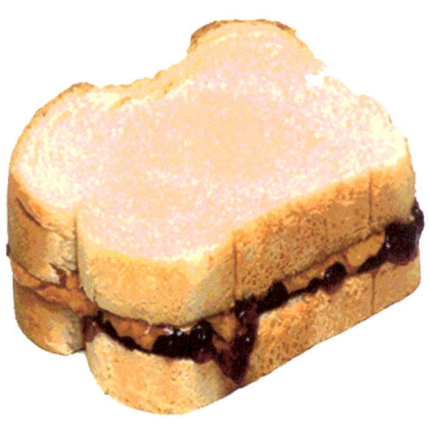

Rest

Event for the Day

Go out produce shopping. Produce is colorful and smells good and there are new faces to see. This all stimulates the senses and it's great for someone who has been in the house all day.

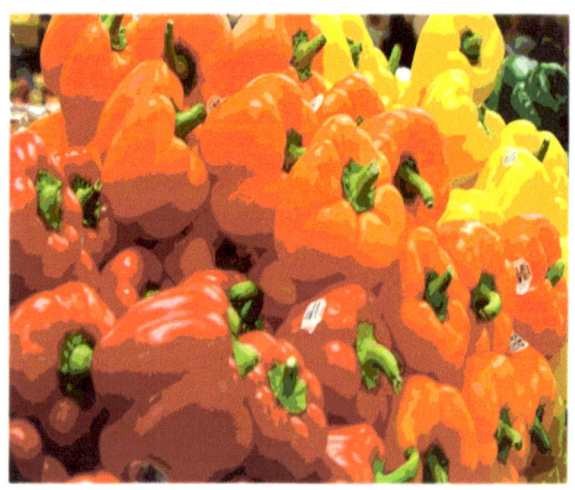

16.

Art Project

Put on some music and begin the project. It can be as simple as cutting out pictures from a magazine and glueing them on to paper to make a collage.

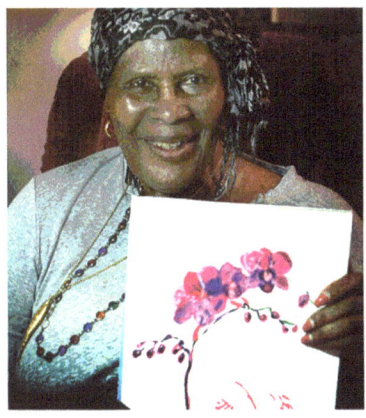

Watch Television

Watch the evening news together and discuss current event and the weather.

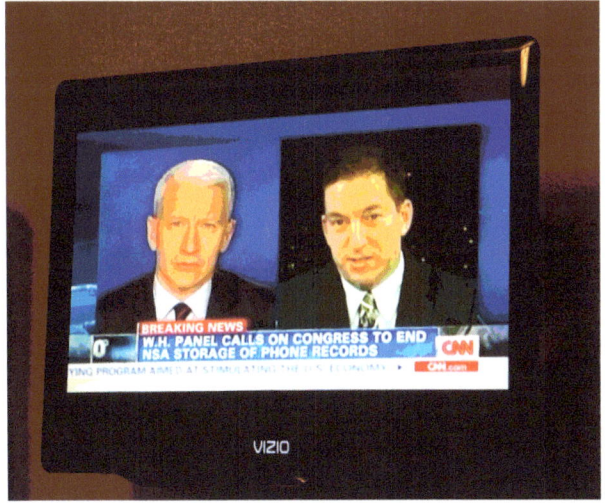

Before Bed

Give your client some tea and aroma therapy before bed.

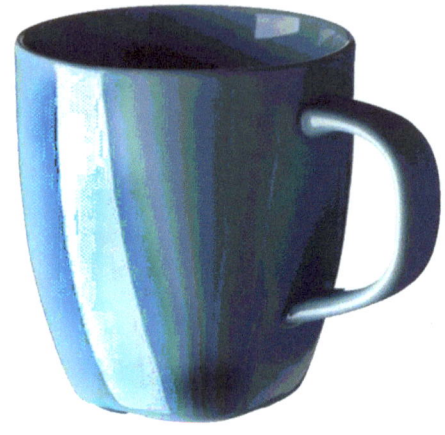

Be Your Client's Best Friend!

Put their needs before your own. Be their advocate. Love yourself for doing such great work and love your client too.

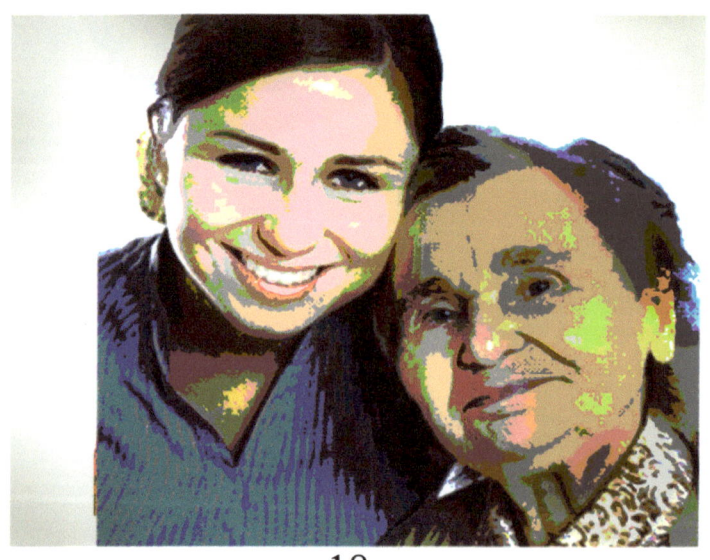

Eat Dinner

Eat dinner together.
It's very lonely to eat by one's self.
Eating together bring people closer together.

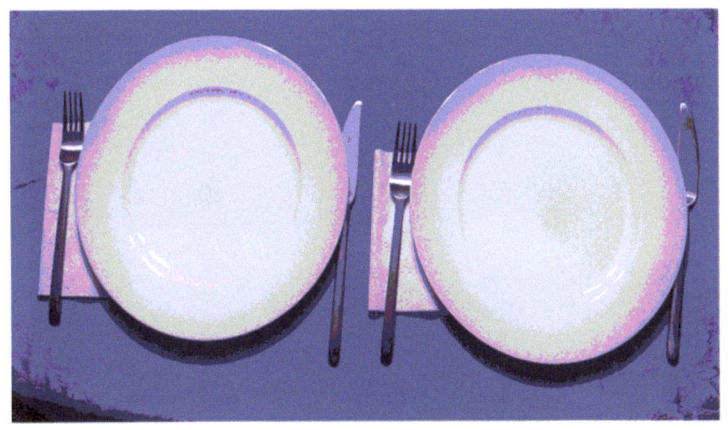

Phone your Client's Family

Help your client to make a phone call to family or friends and tell them about your day.

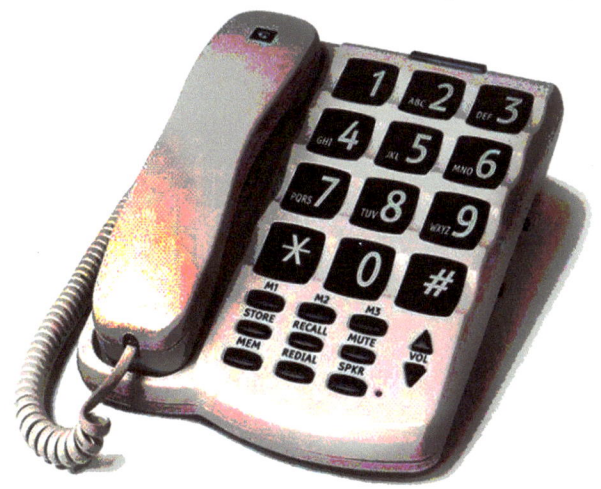

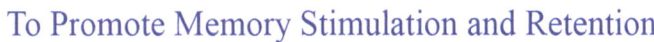

100 Words a Day
Picture flash cards
of everyday common objects

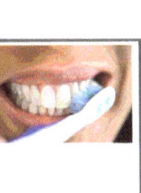

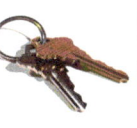

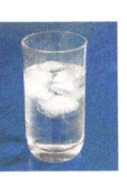

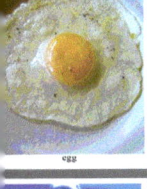

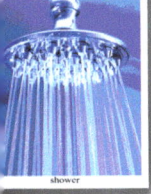

To Promote Memory Stimulation and Retention

Use these flash cards daily and over time they may increase memory retention. They can be used with the word and connect the word with the image. Or simply put you finger over the word and ask, "What is this?" If the user cannot remember, uncover your finger and let him read the word. When he says the word, respond with praise.

To Promote Speech and Conversation Skills
Use the cards as they come out of the box.
The first card is "sunrise".
Show the card and say, "OK You wake up."
Ask, "What do You do first?", Show the picture of the bed and wait for the answer. Then, "you put on your," and show the picture of the slippers. Give a hint! Help the user to get it right and parise them.
Keep asking questions and keep showing pictures.

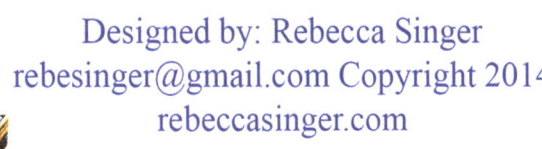

Designed by: Rebecca Singer
rebesinger@gmail.com Copyright 2014
rebeccasinger.com

www.ingramcontent.com/pod-product-compliance
Lightning Source LLC
Chambersburg PA
CBHW041616180526
45159CB00002BC/889